Weight Loss Secrets

PNgFitfam Masterclass Diet 101 Lesson Manual

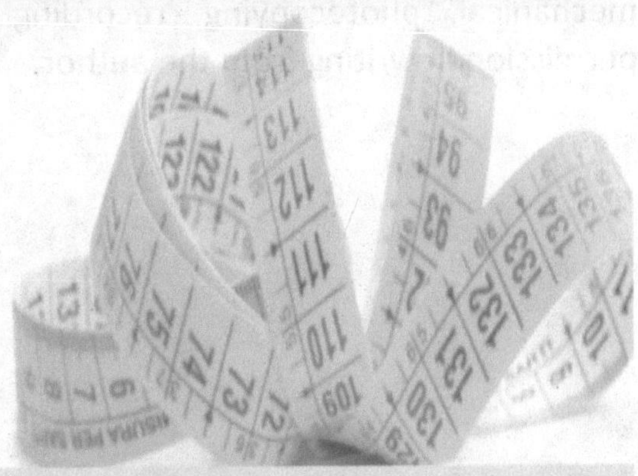

DR NGOZI AWA IMAGA

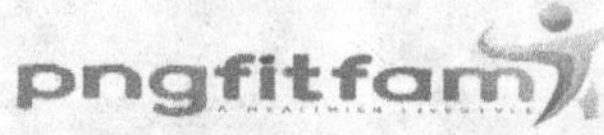

© Dr. Ngozi Imaga

Copyright © November 2019

Preface

This Manual contains TEN lessons to be used over a two-week study period and used as a handy reference book during any of PNgfitfam weight loss programs. At the end of which a Class Quiz will be given and clients assessed on their weight goal progress. Graduation from the program is done once client has achieved their ideal body weight goal. Please study well and do the Activity sections after each lesson.

Dr. Ngozi Imaga
pngfitfamdiet@gmail.com; dr.ngozi@pngfitfam.com
https://pngfitfam.com/; **+234-8094503658**

TABLE OF CONTENTS

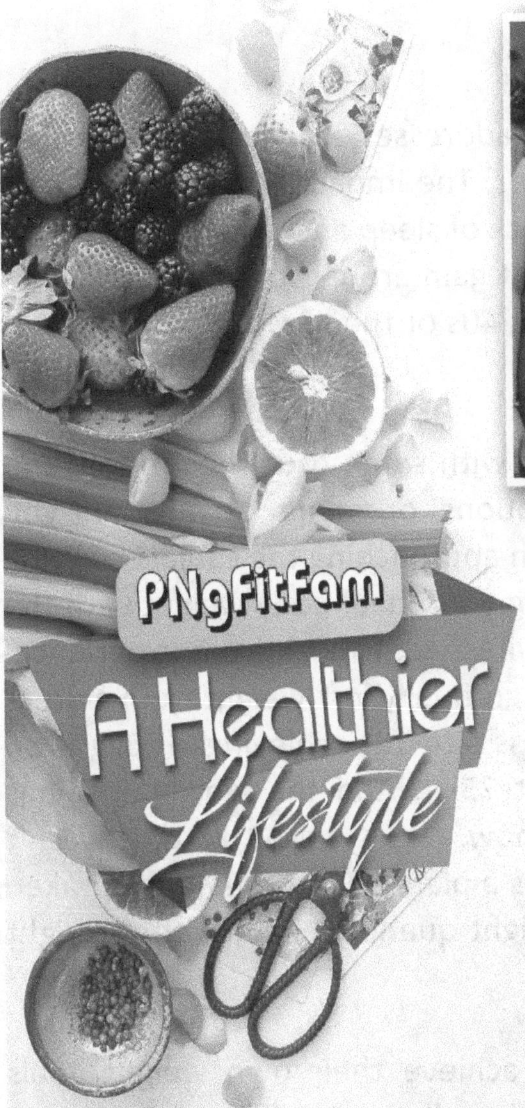

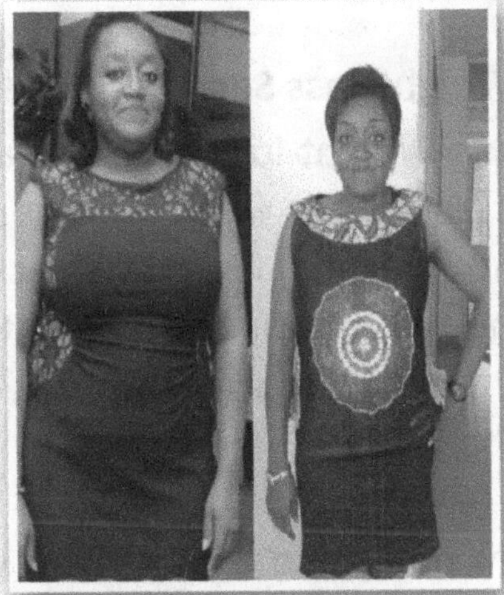

Customized meal plans

Health Guide

Fitness plan

Weight loss diet

Contact details
0809-450-3658
pngfitfam@gmail.com
http://bit.ly/PNgFitFam

Facebook: pngfitfam
Instagram : @pngfitfam

INTRODUCTION

'Weight-loss Secrets'

This Weight-loss program addresses a delicate subject that affects us as we grow older. The impact of food, childbirth, motherhood, life stress, lack of sleep and aging on the body; the tell-tale signs of weight gain around the midsections as one gets into the infamous 40s or the life long struggle with obesity.

I'm not going to bore you with some usual health talk and body mass index calculations or some other stuff you probably already know. I'm approaching the subject of living long and well and attaining your ideal body weight with the right meals and an active lifestyle. I speak from experience. In the space of 8 months I gradually lost weight from a dress size 20 to my current dress size 12, achieving a 20kg drop from 95kg to my present 75kg. And the weight lost has stayed off for two years now. No, it wasn't keto, it wasn't some other fad diet. It was a planned out meal table, taken at the right time, in the right quantities and with the right eating mindset.

I started helping people achieve their own weight goals recently in something I called 'PNgfitfam Diet 101 Masterclass' and the results have been mind blowing. I have designed meal plans for many and placed them in my weightloss programs.

I would like to share with you some **lessons** I taught them along the way that will be useful to you if you want to lose weight or maintain an ideal weight using any of my meal plans. Enjoy!

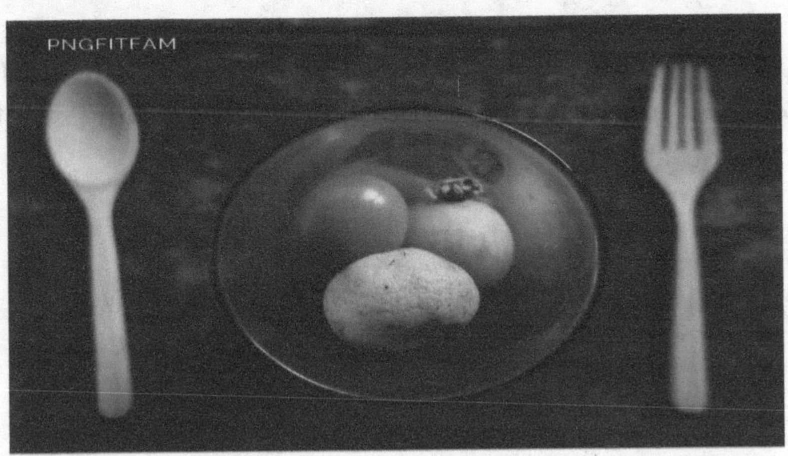

Sign up for the
3 Day Detox Plan

Learn how to school and re-school your tongue to enjoy
healthy food options and rid your body of harmful food toxins.

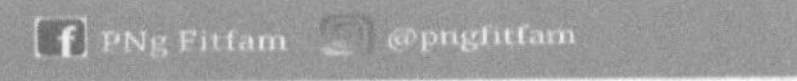

Get Started Today
Visit - bit.ly/PNgFitFam

PNg Fitfam   @pngfitfam

THERE IS NO SUCH TERM AS CHEAT DAY AT PNgfitfam

Yes! All foods are allowed. We have lost all labels. No food is forbidden. However, the portion size and time of day of eating these foods is the culprit.

The foods in your kitchen and fridge and all around you have to be the type that will encourage healthy eating. That way you won't 'cheat'.

And If you do eat something fattening then you do your damage control and not give up, get back in line.

Statistics show that people on a so-called diet tend to think that they are being denied something and this is the major reason they abandon ship at the sight of their greatest food temptation.

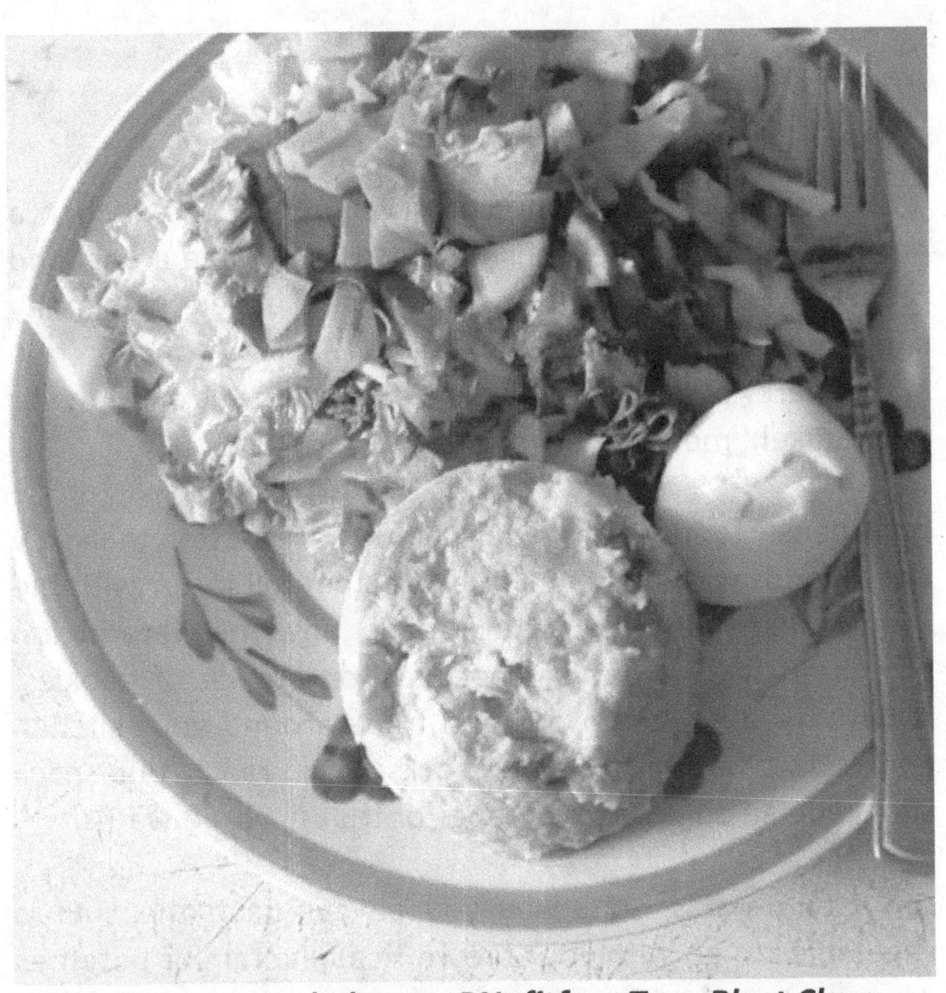

A 12noon meal plate at PNgfitfam Tum-Blast Class

Lesson 2:
CRUSHING THE JUNK FOOD HABIT

'PREP your food'. Meaning you should enter the kitchen a day before or on weekends (in electricity stable areas) and prepare your meals for the day/week ahead in healthy combos and then take to work daily. That way you won't be at the mercy of what we call 'junk' food/pastries or oily/over salty 'bukah' meals.

High dense foods with lower calories are better than low dense foods with higher calories. You get full faster with the former than with the latter. e.g. a bowl of watermelon compared with a bar of chocolate or a pack of cookies. Always have healthy foods and fruits around your kitchen and fridge, not fatty, salty snacks. Your reach out snack should be an apple, some grapes or fruit flavored water.

Learn to do this, that way you always have the cut up vegetables to go with your brown rice, plantain or potatoes when it's time for it.

1. **LIST 10 OF YOUR FAVORITE FOODS BELOW AND USE THE CALORIE COUNTER TO PLACE THEM IN DESCENDING ORDER OF ENERGY**

________________________   ________________________

________________________   ________________________

________________________   ________________________

________________________   ________________________

________________________   ________________________

2. **SUGGEST 3 WAYS YOU CAN PREP YOUR MEALS FOR WORK EACH DAY**

____

____

____

Lesson 3:
BODY TYPES

There are three types of body metabolic dispositions:

The ectomorph: who always seems to "eat a horse" and still remain thin.

The mesomorphs: the upbeat fellow who burns off an equivalent amount of calories taken in with an efficient metabolic profile and loves to exercise.

The endormorphs: those whose body likes to store almost everything they eat in the adipose tissue (fat cells) and don't easily burn off calories. They must be careful of their food intake and the time of the day and the accompanying foods and herbs that will help speed up metabolism and encourage calorie burn even when not at the gym.

It's my desire to move us from being 80% endormorphs to a 50:50 mesomorph - ectomorph body type.

Keep reading this and you too will be posting your "Before and After" pictures soon.

ACTIVITY:

1. Record your 'before' picture today; full snapshot in a fitted dress

2. Go to our pngfitfam Facebook page and post your 'before' look

3. Look out for a gym nearby and register for their aerobics class

4. Clear out the clutter in your kitchen, fridge and dining table

5. Make a new shopping list using the calorie foods guide document

6. Buy a weighing scale and climb it every morning, record the trend

7. Buy a skipping rope and a knee guard if knees are weak; skip daily

8. Log in your breakfast, lunch and dinner in the journal page

9. Visit the@pngfitfam instagram page regularly for updates and inspirational posts

Lesson 4:
FOOD SWAPS

Wheat bread or toasted white bread has lower calories than white bread. Biscuits can work if the oatmeal biscuit type. Vegetable crackers and Hob nobs are also passable. Don't do the cream chocolate biscuits.

Look at the ingredients bar and rule out those with sodium (salt) content more than 2g. Salt taken in excess of this recommended daily allowance will cause your body to retain more water and this will increase your weight on the scale.

Choose boiled foods over fried most of the time. e.g.
*   boiled potatoes over fried potatoes * boiled unripe plantain over fried plantain.
*   Brown rice or quinoa instead of white rice.
*   Beans porridge garnished with vegetables rather than just the oily porridge.
*   Edikaikong/okro/efo riro soup instead of egusi, banga, oily soups.
*   Choose coconut oil over groundnut oil. Make less oily food choices.

MAKE A LIST OF YOUR OWN FOOD SWAPS TO GUIDE YOUR CHOICES

INSTEAD OF WHITE RICE AND STEW	I'LL TAKE BROWN RICE AND FISH STEW

Lesson 5:
STOMACH HUNGER VERSUS MOUTH HUNGER

For those who feel like snacking soon after a meal or in between meals, please don't eat another meal.

A handful of grapes or nuts may just be what you need to quench that transient hunger feeling called mouth hunger. You can even deny gratification and within 20mins the feeling will pass.

But if you don't get full with a meal, then your stomach will still cry out for more.

So, the trick is to enjoy your main meals when you take them and you won't crave for another meal until the appropriate meal time.

The figure on the next page shows you how to control your eating time and habits within a particular eating window. More on this in the next lessons.

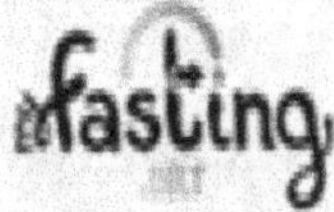

Before 10 am

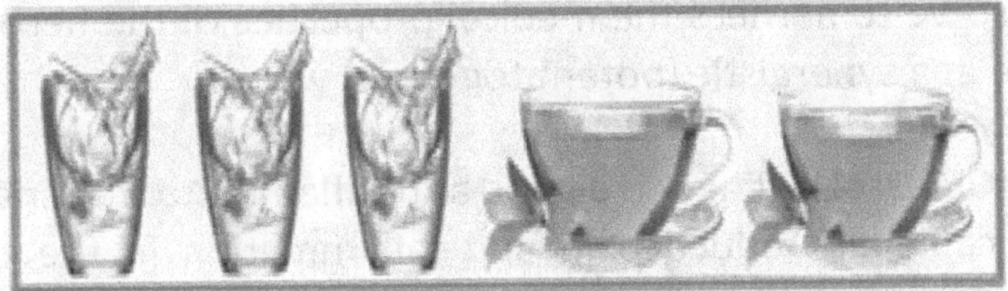

10am - 7 pm

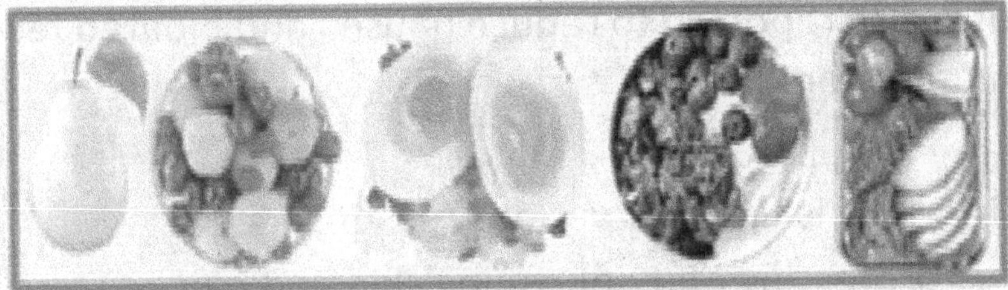

After 7 pm

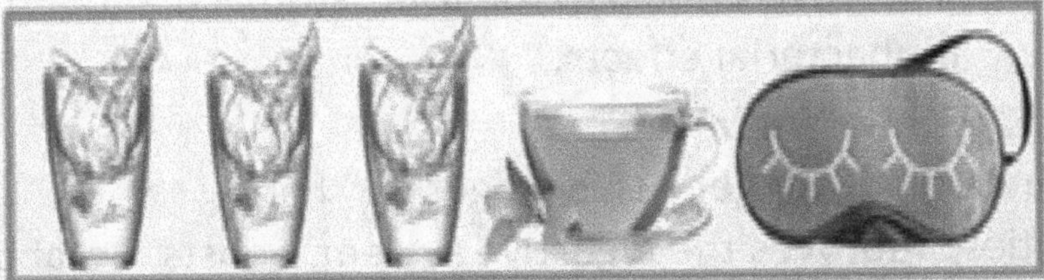

HERBS AND TEAS AS METABOLIC BOOSTERS

Ginger on its own has enormous benefits. Moringa too has been found to have health benefits. Taken in combination will serve to harness the medical properties of the herb and spice in a synergistic (potent together) way.

1. Gingerol in ginger is a good anti-inflammatory agent and can help reduce pain and inflammation in the body when taken.

2. It is also reported to reduce nausea and bloated feelings in the stomach.

3. Moringa is used for various reasons:
   - protecting and nourishing skin and hair.
   - Treating edema (fluid retention).
   - Protective effects in the liver, stomach and also has antibacterial effects.

Moringa and Ginger used together harnesses all these qualities, improves the digestive system, boosts metabolism and nourishes your body.

Caveat on Ginger and Moringa:

If you are on antidiabetic/hypoglycemic or antihypertensive medications please do not co-administer with moringa. It has been known to lower blood sugar levels. This is great for after meal times when sugar levels spike. But not good if you are already taking drugs to do that. The combination could be lethal.

Also, those who are pregnant are not advised to take ginger because of its mild abortifacient (causing miscarriage) properties. It can bring on an early cycle. Having said that, note that 1 tea bag quantity as suggested earlier is relatively safe for use.

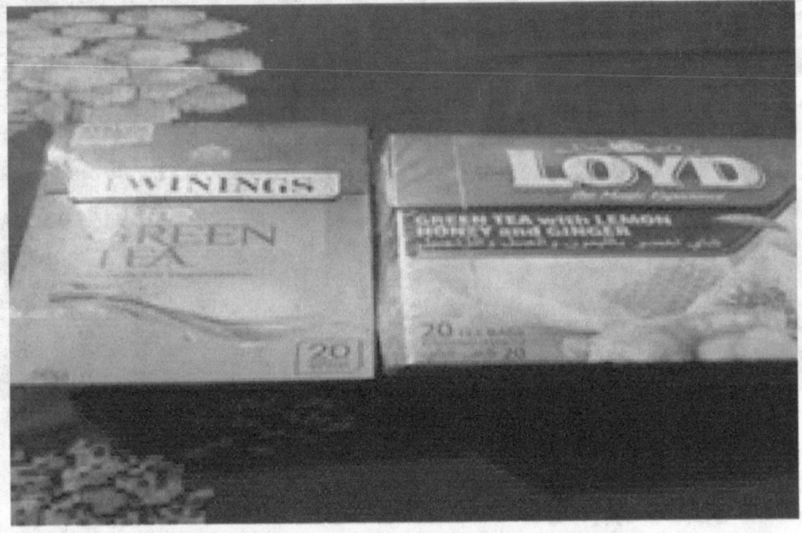

Green Tea varieties: fat burners.

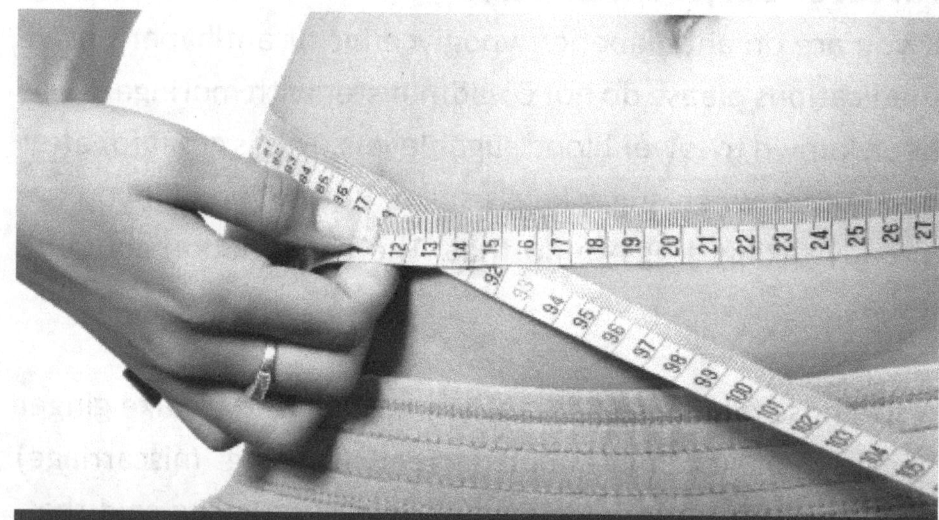

HERE AT PNGFITFAM, WE MAKE SURE TO CREATE A DIET PLAN THAT SUITS YOU AND YOUR BODY. REACH YOUR GOALS WITH US!

Lesson 7:

BELLY FAT BURNERS/TUMMY BLASTER

Forget Tummy tuck surgery or waist trimmer! These foods help you burn belly fat and lose weight fast: Yogurt, whole grains, berries, flax seeds and ofcourse water.

These are low fat and low calorie foods that help combat bloating, speed up metabolism and reduce insulin and cortisol levels in the body.

Meals rich in Protein (plant protein), legumes, avocados, cucumber-lemon-ginger mix, apple cider are all metabolic boosters that have a wholesome impact on your tummy in synergy with tummy exercises.

To lose belly fat there are a few things to consider.

Balance your macronutrients: carbohydrates, protein, and fat. we need all three in our diet.

Carbohydrates: provide fuel, the energy for your body and brain. it's found in all plant foods, like grains, fruits, vegetables, and legumes but typically stay away from grains and get your carbs by eating fruit, veggies, and legumes.

Protein: helps to build and repair your muscles, organs, skin, blood, and different chemicals, like hormones, in your body. it's found in meat, poultry, fish, legumes, dairy (milk and Greek yogurt), tofu, and eggs, and in smaller amounts in nuts, seeds, and whole grains.

Fat: insulates and protects your bones and organs, acts as a backup fuel for energy, and helps in brain development.

Healthy, unsaturated fats: are found in olive oil, avocados, nuts, seeds, and fatty fish, like salmon, sardines, and mackerel. unhealthy saturated fats are found in high-fat beef, pork, butter, full-fat dairy, and processed foods, like cookies and donuts.

Please stay away from processed foods as they are high in sugar. consuming too much sugar increases weight gain and leads to belly fat.

DIET AND EXERCISE GO TOGETHER

For the healthy meal plans or belly fat burners to work, it has to be combined with aerobics and abs (abdominal) exercises.

Register at a gym or get a good Trainer to coach you. Your weight loss effort is 80% diet and 20% exercise. Each one has its place. So be open to this.

Good sleep is essential for weight loss. There must be periods of rest after workout so that the effects can impact on body cells and so that your tissues can be restored.

For many years, we've been told to cut calories and exercise more right?! wrong.

While exercise is key to staying active our diet is the most important factor to living well and very long in strength and healthy.

The place of the skipping rope cannot be over emphasized. It helped me immensely to lose weight and now helps to regulate my weight.

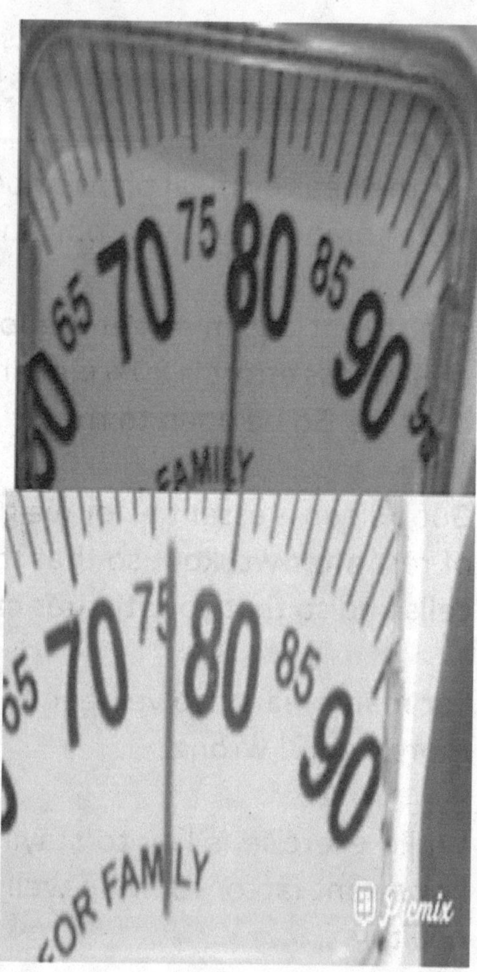

skipping session. 2kg off

Lesson 9:

INTERMITTENT FASTING

This is really quite simple and helps our bodies get into fat-burning mode. A simple form of intermittent fasting limits the hours of the day when you eat. Typically, your first meal is consumed around noon and the last meal before eight which means you have an eight-hour window to eat your meals. By limiting nighttime eating your overnight fast is extended which significantly benefits your metabolism.

Here are some benefits of intermittent fasting:

A. Reducing levels of insulin, which makes it easier for the body to use stored fat.

B. Lowering blood sugars, blood pressure, and inflammation levels.

C. Changing the expression of certain genes, which helps the body protect itself from disease as well as promoting longevity.

D. Dramatically increases human growth hormone, or HGH, which helps the body utilize body fat and grow muscle.

The body activates a healing process doctors call autophagy, which essentially means that the body digests or recycles old or damaged cell components.

Lesson 10:

METABOLIC CONFUSION

The previous lesson on metabolic body type refers. Are you an endormorph, mesomorph or ectomorph? Please read it again (Lesson 3).

Metabolic Confusion has to do with calorie confusion or carbs cycling.

What is Calorie Cycling? Calorie cycling, also called calorie shifting, is a dieting style that allows you to cycle between low-calorie and higher calorie periods.
So a reduction in total calorie intake is recommended to lose weight.

However, more is not always better. Cutting too many calories can actually hurt your ability to lose weight and keep it off. ... If we restrict calories (energy), then the body has to slow down to preserve energy, which means our metabolism slows down. That's why I have designed alternate days of eating well/not eating 'well' in my meal plan. Adhere to the cycles. Don't just eat one type of way each day.

When you starve or restrict diet everyday, the body conserves the little energy it gets and thereby prevents weightloss and no downward incline on the scale. That's not

19

what we want. So take the metabolic boosters/teas daily and work that meal plan and rock your scale.

Accountability to the weighing scale
Unlike what most people think, climbing the same scale at the same time the day (first thing in the morning after bowel movement and before any drink of water) with the same minimal clothing, is a sure way of testing your progress and evaluating the impact of the previous day's meal and activity level. It personally helps me stay on course and crush all bad eating habits.

Finally,

Discipline and Determination are catalysts for self-motivation
The intermittent fasting 16:8 eating window, the composition of your food plate and food quantity play a combined role in weight management.

The foods and juices you forgo, the taste buds and sweet tooth denials and the drive to be better and do better than your yesterday are key factors to the results you want to achieve/maintain.

If you are already on a Weight loss journey, don't relax otherwise the weight will come back so fast and so much you will be amazed.

Weight loss as I am teaching and showing you is about what, when and how you eat. Some nutrition psychology and biochemistry expertise is communicated to you in all my lessons so that your victory is a permanent one.

Keep at it. Be dogged in your determination.

Let the scales concur (or not), let your clothing size show you your progress (or not) .... You just keep doing what you've been told to do here. Follow a healthy meal plan, do your skipping and exercises and sleep well at night. I'm rooting for you over here!

Welcome to the healthier lifestyle!

Contact me for your meal plan design and weight evaluation
Dr Ngozi Awa Imaga
CEO PNgfitfam,
Nutritional and Pharmacological Biochemist
pngfitfamdiet@gmail.com; +234-8094503658

TESTIMONIALS FROM CLIENTS

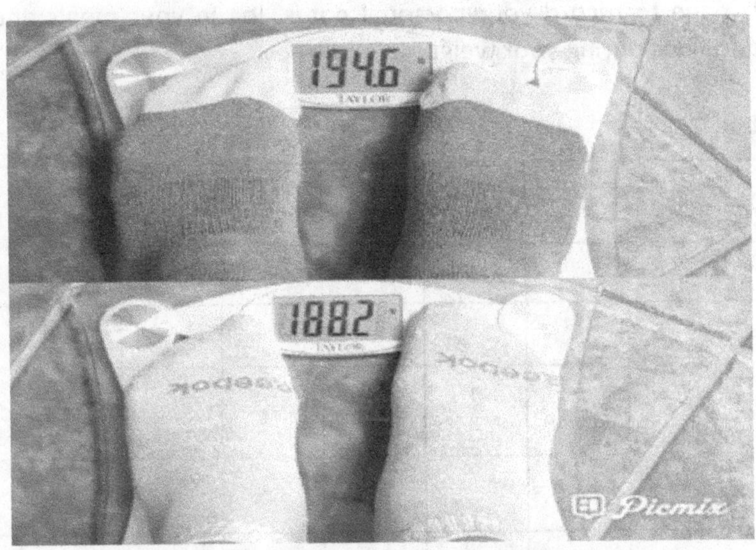

Client On Day 9, Steadily Making Progress, losing 3kg/6 pounds within a week!

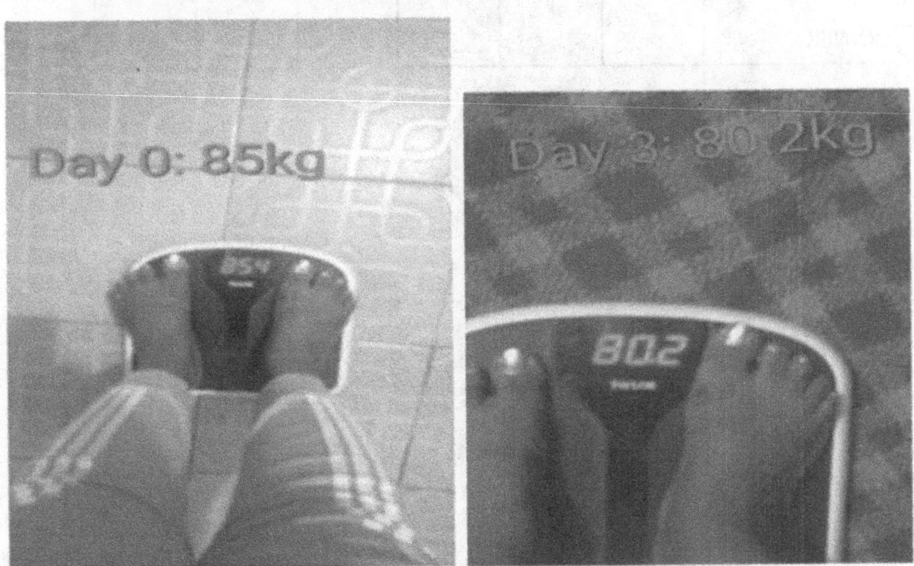

Client On Day 3 Tum-Blast Plan, Making landslide Progress. Losing 5kg in 3 days

PERSONAL JOURNAL

Use this page to record your personal notes, log in your meals and make active decisions during your weight loss journey.

WEEK 1

ACTIVITY	DAY 1	DAY 2	DAY 3	DAY 4	DAY 5	DAY 6	DAY 7
WEIGHT:							
WAISTLINE:							
NUMBER OF SKIPS DONE:							
BREAKFAST:							
LUNCH							
DINNER							
ACTION NOTES							

WEEK 2

ACTIVITY	DAY 1	DAY 2	DAY 3	DAY 4	DAY 5	DAY 6	DAY 7
WEIGHT:							
WAISTLINE:							
NUMBER OF SKIPS DONE:							
BREAKFAST:							
LUNCH							
DINNER							
ACTION NOTES							

WEEK 3

ACTIVITY	DAY 1	DAY 2	DAY 3	DAY 4	DAY 5	DAY 6	DAY 7
WEIGHT:							
WAISTLINE:							
NUMBER OF SKIPS DONE:							
BREAKFAST:							
LUNCH							
DINNER							
ACTION NOTES							

WEEK 4

ACTIVITY	DAY 1	DAY 2	DAY 3	DAY 4	DAY 5	DAY 6	DAY 7
WEIGHT:							
WAISTLINE:							
NUMBER OF SKIPS DONE:							
BREAKFAST:							
LUNCH							
DINNER							
ACTION NOTES							

PNgFitfam Healthy Food swaps
MEAL TABLE (Nigerian foods)

Wake up: Drink 25cl of water (room Temp)

7am to 10am: No food. just Water/Green Tea/Coffee/Lemon mix Eating window: 10am to 7 pm

Daily calories: 2,000 - 2,400kcal

DAY	BREAKFAST - 10am max	LUNCH - 3pm max	SNACK 12pm or 5pm	DINNER - 7pm max
1	A serving of fruit Quaker oats - 3 tablespoons Akara Akara balls 2 med. size	Brown rice - One serving spoon and stew with steamed vegetables (1 cup)	Tiger nuts or Grapes - a handful	Fish pepper soup (small bowl) 1 Boiled unripe plantain
2	Momoi - 2 medium sized wraps Guinea corn pap - 2 serving spoons	1 portion Vegetable salad (Cucumber, Cabbage, lettuce, broccoli) Fried fish - 1 pc	2 Garden eggs with peanut paste	Beans plantain porridge -2 spoons with spinach (handful)
3.	Quaker oats - 3 tablespoons w/water Fried green plantain - 1 stick	1 Roasted unripe plantain with stew and 2 boiled eggs	Boiled groundnut or walnuts - 1 handful	1 small bowl of Vegetable soup with 1 fist size wheat meal
4	Momoi - 2 medium sized wraps Guinea corn pap - 2 serving spoons	Okra/vegetable soup 2 serving spoons with wheat - 1 fist size	Coconut/Nigerian pear - 1	3 slices of boiled Sweet Potatoes and 1 spoon of cooked beans with stew
5	2 slices of wheat bread with half an avocado as spread and a cup of ginger tea	2 serving spoons of Chicken sauce and Quinoa or brown or basmati rice (1/4 cup)	lemonade drink - 25cl	2 serving spoons of Afang/Edikaikong soup with wheat or unripe plantain or oatmeal (1 fist size)
6	2 medium size Akara balls , 1 small bowl of Guinea corn pap	half a medium size Sweet potato and fish stew	Unsweetened yoghurt - 20cl	A large bowl of vegetable salad without cream 1 grilled piece chicken
7	1 Boiled unripe plantain, one boiled egg and fish stew	Vegetable/Efo riro soup - 2 serving spoons with wheat - 1 fist size	Grape flavored water - 1 glass	1/2 cup of Brown rice and 1 spoon of chicken sauce

INSTRUCTIONS FOR WEIGHTLOSS

1. Drink Water Always
2. **SPICES:** Use turmeric, ginger, garlic, black pepper seasonings to cook most meals.
3. **A SERVING OF FRUIT DAILY:** Apple, purple grapes, plums, Avocados. These have low glycemic index. Do less of pineapples or bananas if weight loss is your desire.
4. Get used to these meal patterns on the table. choose boiled foods over fried. stay away from oily soups, white rice or white bread.
5. For week 1 - Eat as advised in the table chart above
6. From week 2: reduce your daily meals to just 2 of those listed. preferably morning and dinner foods. skip lunch. Take water instead at lunchtime.
7. By week 4: Eat just the lunch listings and skip breakfast and dinner. replace those times with water/green tea/ginger and garlic mix/cucumber and carrot slices.
8. Apply the 16 hour fast and 8 hour eating rule. this method of intermittent fasting will get you your results quicker.
9. At the end of this first four weeks, you will be ready for a more aggressive weight loss plan at a 1,400kcal maximum daily calorie intake.

Contact me and pay for the Phase II weight-loss specific plans when ready and kick off your fitness journey with gusto.

Give me feedback on your progress.

Welcome to the healthy lifestyle!

-Dr. Ngozi Imaga

Nutritional Biochemist and CEO, PNgFitfam
pngfitfamdiet@gmail.com; https://pngfitfam.com